# Ketogenic Diet: Ketogenic Diet Mistakes to Avoid for Rapid Weight Loss

By Dan Tucker

# Table of Contents

**Mistake #16: Neglecting MCTs**
**Conclusion**
**Cheat Sheet**

# Introduction

Society is slowly realizing that so-called 'conventional wisdom' has health and dieting completely wrong. For decades on end, it was generally accepted that carbohydrates were good and fat was bad, period. Cementing this incorrect notion was the fact that the food pyramid had grains, wheat, and foods high in carbohydrates featured prominently at its base.

Recently, however, science has begun to show that when it comes to a healthy diet, it is actually the exact opposite that's true. In other words, carbohydrates are bad and fat is good!

This societal realization has led to the revival of many diets advocating variations of a low-carb and high-fat (LCHF) intake. Among these diets, one of the most prominent is, of course, the ketogenic diet.

The ketogenic diet has become hugely popular, not because it's a fad (it's not), but because it delivers astounding results. Furthermore, it's benefits appeal to a surprisingly diverse selection of people.

It's used by those seeking to lose weight and get it shape. It's used by bodybuilders seeking to gain muscle. It's used by top athletes seeking to improve their performance. It's used by CEOs and entrepreneurs seeking to boost mental clarity and concentration. Heck, it's even used to stop epilepsy and has been shown to prevent strokes, Parkinson's disease, Alzheimer's disease, and more!

Nonetheless, many struggle to actualize the abundant benefits of the ketogenic diet. Whether they struggle to achieve ketosis and conclude that "it doesn't work" for them, or they have difficulty maintaining ketosis, or results seem to plateau, they fail to reap the rewards they desire and deserve.

If that's you and you were beginning to lose hope, you're in luck!

There are many common misconceptions and mistakes that prevent people from reaping the full benefits of the ketogenic diet, and if you've fallen prey to these errors, you're not alone. The key to overcoming these issues, reaping the full rewards of ketosis, and becoming a fat-burning machine is *knowledge*. Knowing *how* to get it working for you. The process, the biochemistry, and the easily avoidable mistakes.

In fact, according to Dr. Jeff S. Volek and Dr. Stephen D. Phinney — two of the world's leading researchers on low-carb diets — there are many mistakes people make that lead to suboptimal results. Through the countless studies they've conducted and the thousands of patients they've treated, they've found that there are some common stumbling blocks that ketogenic dieters run into.

These common mistakes prevent people from getting into full-blown ketosis and reaping all of the metabolic benefits.

To discover what you're doing wrong and how to easily fix these mistakes, read on!

# Mistake #1: Scale Surveillance

When you're on a diet, it can be hugely tempting to plop yourself onto the scale each morning and use that as a sign of your progress. The only problem with this is that the number on the scale is a poor indicator of your health or progress.

In fact, some people I know have actually seen their weight *increase* when on the ketogenic diet.

Wait, what?!

That's right, they *gained* weight. Not because they became fatter, but because they gained muscle. Their body fat percentage dropped while their lean muscle mass increased. More specifically, they actually lost eight pounds of fat and gained nine pounds of muscle. In other words, they lost almost 10 pounds of fat in just under six weeks, but gained weight.

Beginning to see while scales are the least important metric you can use when gauging your success?

If my friend in the example had been obsessing over the number on the scale, she would have concluded that the ketogenic diet made her fatter when, in reality, just the opposite was true.

Meanwhile, many people starve themselves on lettuce-leaf "diets." This forces their body in starvation mode where it breaks down muscle for energy, as muscle is a richer and more easily accessible source of energy than fat. It also stores *more* fat for future use (as the body thinks it is starving). As a result, they lose muscle mass while the fat remains virtually untouched. They then jump onto the scales, see that their total weight has decreased, and feel that they have succeed. In reality, however, their decrease in weight is the result of a loss of muscle, not fat. They remain just as unhealthy, if not more so.

So even though my friend technically gained a little weight, she found herself showered in compliments on how fit she looked. She had replaced unwanted fat with lean muscle.

The hard truth is that scales just tells you that you have a certain amount of bone, tissue, and water inside of you. Not very useful when it comes to losing fat.

Imagine a small room with a scale inside. On the door, there is a screen that tells you the weight of the person inside. But you can't see who it actually is standing on the scales.

First up, the scale reads "250 lbs." Everybody outside the room gasps, wondering how the person even managed to fit inside the small room. They imagine a morbidly obese person inside.

Then the door opens, and bodybuilder Arnold Schwarzenegger swaggers out.

Although an extreme example, it illustrates the point. You could have a people of the same height and weight, and one looks a little chubby while the other looks slim, fit, and toned.

You cannot hold the number on the scale in such high regard. The scale lies. It doesn't tell you the whole truth. Losing weight is not the same as losing fat.

If you want to know whether or not you're losing fat, a scale won't help. Instead, you can measure the circumference of your weight with a measuring tape, have your body fat percentage checked each month, take pictures, ask yourself how you feel, if you have more energy, how your clothes fit, and so on.

# Mistake #2: Protein Problems

Protein is arguably the most important macro. Compared to other macronutrients, it increases fat burning. This means that generally, more protein leads to weight loss, muscle gain, and improved body composition. That's why you often see bodybuilders drinking their macho protein shakes and raw egg drinks (egg is rich in protein).

That being said, too much protein can end up sabotaging your efforts to reach ketosis. This happens because 56 percent of protein can be converted to glucose. So by eating way more protein than your body needs, you leave excess protein. This excess protein is then converted into glucose, which prevents your body from going into full-blown ketosis.

The aim of the ketogenic diet is to make the body rely on fat, rather than glucose, for energy. Foods high in carbohydrates are eliminated for this reason, as carbohydrates are converted into glucose, which the body then uses for energy. Similarly, though, if you have too much protein, the body converts it into glucose. This glucose is then used for energy, rather than fat, which prevents ketosis.

Many people on the ketogenic diet find that in the beginning they drop lots of weight (mostly water). Eventually, however, their body levels off to around 1–2 pounds per week. If you find yourself plateauing (or struggling to achieve or maintain ketosis), you should definitely take a look at your protein intake.

After all, the purpose of the ketogenic diet is to make fat your main source of energy. When you eat carbs or have excess protein, your body derives its energy from glucose, preventing ketosis.

To achieve ketosis, it is generally advised that 70–75 percent of your calories come from fat, 20–25 percent from protein, and five percent from carbohydrates.

The experts agree on this, too. According to Dr. Jeff S. Volek and Dr. Stephen D. Phinney (the world leading low-carb diet researchers mentioned earlier), a "well-formulated" low-carb diet should be high in fat, moderate in protein, and — obviously — low in carbohydrates.

The key takeaway is that protein intake should be *moderate*. When it comes to protein, a good range to aim for is 0.7–0.9 grams per pound of bodyweight, or 1.5–2.0 grams per kilogram of bodyweight.

So, for example, if you weigh 70 kilograms or 154 pounds, that is between 105–140 grams of protein.

All in all, protein can be converted into glucose and so too much protein can prevent you from getting into ketosis.

# Mistake #3: Crazy for Carbs

A major mistake that many make when trying to achieve ketosis is eating too many carbs. Even though you might think that you're eating hardly any carbs, it's not uncommon for people to not realize just how many carbs they're consuming.

After all, carbohydrates are not only found in grains.

You had two bananas today? That's 50 grams of carbohydrates, enough to potentially prevent ketosis.

You been snacking on nuts all day long at work? Eating lots of nuts, such as almonds and cashews, can increase your carbohydrate intake to a level at which ketosis is either prevented or has suboptimal benefits.

It can be easy to simply stop eating grain-based foods — such as bread, pasta, rice, and cereal — and assume that you've eliminated all carbs from your diet. The reality, however, is that carbs are sneaky and hide in unexpected places. If you're not careful, they can quickly add up without you even realizing and prevent ketosis.

A great tool to instantaneously find out how many carbs are in something is to search, "how many carbs in [food]," on Google. Google has an in-built tool that instantly lets you know, without you needing to open any websites or anything. You can easily do this on your smartphone when out and about.

To achieve ketosis, it is recommended that you have no more than 20–50 grams of carbohydrates. While there are some people that find they can get great results on more, such as 100 grams, this is not sufficient for most people. To get into ketosis and have plenty of ketones flood through your bloodstream and supply your brain with lots of energy, you will almost certainly need to go below 50 grams of carbohydrates per day.

Many people, without realizing, exceed 50 grams per day and fail to achieve ketosis. They then conclude that the ketogenic diet just "doesn't work" for them.

If you want to reap the full metabolic benefits of ketosis, consume less 50 grams of carbohydrates each day. Moreover, if 50 grams doesn't work either, temporarily going under 20 grams can work.

An important thing to note when going under 50 grams a day is that you will need to eliminate most fruits from your diet.

All in all, some people are sensitive to carbohydrates or simply consume too many without realizing (or both!). A good rule of thumb is to eat less than 50 grams of carbohydrates each day.

# Mistake #4: Electrolyte Errors

When you're on the ketogenic diet, electrolyte (salt/sodium) imbalance can be a big deal. A common mistake made by those unfamiliar with the ketogenic diet is to not get enough salt.

This is understandable as we are so used to avoiding salts. However, when you're on the ketogenic diet, your body actually *needs* more salt. Low-carb diets are natriuretic, which means that the kidneys dump sodium.

One of biggest reasons that low-carb diets work so well is that they reduce insulin levels. Insulin is the hormone that helps turn glucose into fat. Insulin also inhibits the production of ketone bodies. As carbohydrates are converted into glucose (which is turned into fat by insulin), a low-carb diet reduces insulin levels.

However, in addition to telling cells to store fat, insulin also tells the kidneys to hold onto sodium. So when you go on an insulin-reducing low-carb diet, your body starts shedding excess sodium.

This sodium deficiency can lead to headaches, dizziness, fatigue, and even constipation. This sodium depletion can then lead to the kidneys starting to excrete potassium in an attempt to conserve sodium, resulting in muscle cramps.

Not getting enough potassium — the electrolyte responsible for proper muscle function — can have significant negative effects. To avoid the resulting muscle cramps and feeling as if you're about to pass out, it's a good idea to take appropriate multivitamins and/or supplements.

Although potassium is naturally found fruits, such as bananas, the ketogenic diet omits most fruits due to their carbohydrate content. Consequently, other forms of it, such as multivitamins and supplements, are generally the only way to make sure that you get enough potassium.

With regards to sodium, make sure to consume 3–5 grams of it each day. You can do this by adding more salt to your foods or drinking a cup of broth. It is also important to drink lots of water as it gets dispelled so quickly.

Conveniently, these solutions also significantly help with the keto flu.

# Mistake #5: Fat Fears

As mentioned earlier, fat should count for 70–75 percent of your intake on the ketogenic diet. To put it simply, that's a hell of a lot of fat.

The problem, though, is that people still have a fear of fat. They've been continuously told ever since they were children that fat is bad. And yes, consuming such quantities of fat would be alarming if one were still eating a typical Western high-carb diet. On the ketogenic diet, however, it is necessary.

Consider it this way: A typical person consumes mostly carbohydrates. Lots of bread, pasta, cereal, rice, and sugary foods. All of these carbohydrates are converted into glucose and used for energy.

On the ketogenic diet, however, carbohydrates are virtually eliminated. Instead, your body derives energy from fat — not glucose. As such, you can think of yourself replacing carbohydrates with fat (which you are!).

Instead of being afraid of piling on the bacon and putting tablespoons of butter, coconut oil, and thick cream into your coffee, just consider it no more unusual than a person having some cereal and toast for breakfast. They're getting their energy from carbohydrates and you're getting your energy from fats.

A mistake that many people make when starting out with the ketogenic diet is that they hold onto their ingrained fear of fatty foods. It's not uncommon for those new to the diet to continue getting foods labeled "low-fat."

While that's understandable after spending a lifetime trying to avoid fat, just trust the ketogenic diet and enjoy the fat. Your body's unique biochemical response to dietary fat in the absence of carbohydrates makes it highly improbable that you can consume too much of it. So eat that full fat cheese, munch all the skin off your chicken, and slather butter all over your broccoli.

Unfortunately, it's also not uncommon for those unfamiliar with the ketogenic diet and the body's inner workings to assume that if low-carb is good, then low-carb *and* low-fat must be even better. To put it simply, this is a *huge* mistake.

If you eliminate both carbohydrates *and* fat, you will literally starve. So when you go low-carb, eliminating carbohydrates as an energy source, you *need* to replace it with something else (i.e. fat).

All of those carbohydrate-rich meals that you've stopped eating since undertaking the ketogenic diet need to be replaced with meals rich in fat. If you don't increase your fat intake in order to compensate, you will end up feeling hungry and terribly unwell and will eventually give up.

Furthermore, there is actually no scientific reason to fear fat — you just need to make sure that you are eating healthy fats. Healthy fats include monounsaturated, saturated, and Omega-3s. Unhealthy fats include vegetable oils and trans fats.

Finally, "low-fat" foods are very high in carbohydrates. They replace the fat that they've taken out with sugar to keep it tasting good. If you are not careful with your eating and make sure to count where your calories are coming from, it can be easy to unknowingly be eating a low-fat, high-carb diet!

So get over your fear of fat and go all in.

All in all, to have enough energy to sustain yourself on a low-carb diet, eat lots and lots of fat. It's not called a low-carb *high-fat* diet for nothing.

# Mistake #6: The Negotiator

Another common reason that people fail with the ketogenic diet is that they are not fully committed.

The reality is that the ketogenic diet is not for the half-hearted. You can't sit on the fence. You *must* commit. You *must* have determination and grit. You *must* be all in.

Not fully committing and instead remaining somewhere between high-carb and high-fat is a disastrous — not to mention dangerous — combination.

When it comes to the ketogenic diet, don't try to negotiate. Don't tell yourself, "Well, eating this will only keep me out of ketosis for a few days, but then I'll get right back on track!" Don't try to eat burnt toast so that your body can't digest the carbs.

Anything less than total commitment will result in failure.

There are millions of delicious meals that you can eat on the ketogenic diet. If you have to regularly eat meals that you know will kick you out of ketosis, or if you have to eat burnt toast, then you are obviously not fully committed to reaping the rewards and achieving your health goals.

You must either be all out or all in. You can't be both.

# Mistake #7: Fake Food

The ketogenic diet is about more than just lowering your carbohydrate intake. You need to eat *real* food — real, nutritious foods. Not the likes of dodgy Atkins bars or Quest bars, they are processed foods. They're not real food and they're not good for you.

Eat ingredients (i.e. there is no food, just the ingredients that make food!), not the sort of stuff that comes in individual wrappers.

So stick to the ingredients. Vegetables, eggs, meats, fish, and healthy fats.

Also, stick away from so-called "low-carb" products. Processed foods labeled "low-carb" are almost always much higher in carbs than they would have you believe and often contain unwanted additives.

Likewise, "sugar-free" treats are not as safe as they would have you believe. Most sweet foods contain sugar in the form of fructose, sucrose, or glucose, and are thus high in carbohydrates. As a result, whenever you eat sweet food, your body will expect carbohydrates and will get ready for a carb hit. When no carbs come, it gets confused and you end up with strong cravings for sugar. In addition to the artificial sweeteners, pre-packaged foods are also full of chemicals and preservatives, all of which hinder your weight loss and lead to a plateau.

If you want to get into full-blown ketosis, try to avoid deceptively labeled processed foods as well as pre-prepared meals full of additives.

Eat real food.

# Mistake #8: Friendly Fats and Unfriendly Fats

Another mistake made by would-be fat burners when implementing the ketogenic diet is that they eat the wrong kind of fat. That's right, not all fats are equal. A high-fat diet won't serve you any good — in fact, it will damage your health — if you're eating the wrong kind of fat.

So what are the good fats and what are the bad fats?

Good fats are include saturated fats and monounsaturated fats. These types of fats have a healthy impact on your joints, brain, body fat, cholesterol, and so on.

Bad fats — in addition to sabotaging your ketogenic diet efforts — are highly toxic and lead to increased risk of heart disease, cancer, diabetes, and obesity. Bad fats are trans fats, of which vegetable oils contain massive amounts of.

Foods that contain good fats include avocados, olive oil, coconut oil, nuts, cheese, Greek yogurt, sour cream, heavy whipping cream, butter, and animal fats.

Foods that contain bad fats include margarine, vegetable shortening, vegetable oils, seed oils, and most others not mentioned above with the good fats. It is also worth noting that most processed foods will contain trans fats (i.e. bad fats).

So avoid the bad fats and go all in on the good fats.

# Mistake #9: Flu Fighters

Feeling exhausted, sick, tired, and unwell? Bedridden? 100 percent convinced that the ketogenic diet just isn't for you? That it makes you sick, tired, and just "doesn't work" for you? About to give up on this whole keto thing?

Don't.

When starting out on the ketogenic diet, many people — though not everyone — experience what is known as the "keto flu" during the first few days as their body adapts to burning ketones rather than glucose.

Symptoms include fatigue, sleepiness, nausea,brain fog, an upset stomach, and headaches — hence it's comparison to the flu. You feel sick.

Typically these symptoms last anywhere from a day to a week, though some people don't experience them at all. If you work a normal job, it's best to start ketogenic diet on a weekend or during a time that you're able to deal with the symptoms and get lots of rest.

If you do get a bad bout of the keto flu, don't give up! Get through it and, eventually, you'll find yourself waking up feeling refreshed for the first time in years with a euphoria and energy that persists all day long. No more afternoon slumps! Oh, and you'll also be dropping weight like a B-52 drops bombs.

Keto flu symptoms are caused by the body needing to start producing fat-burning enzymes for energy instead of carbs, which initially poses a bit of dilemma for the body as it had been producing heaps glucose-burning enzymes ready for your next high-carb meal.

Also, as the body is not used to such an influx of fat, diarrhea (or sometimes constipation) is not uncommon. This is yet another reason that it's best to start your ketogenic journey on a weekend — you don't want to be stuck in traffic Tuesday morning on the way to work when the urgent need to get to the closest possible bathroom overcomes you.

All that being said, there are a few things that you can do to help lessen the keto flu symptoms.

Firstly, drink heaps of water. And then some more.

Secondly, as we discussed earlier, going on the ketogenic diet will lead to your kidneys dumping heaps of sodium, causing an electrolyte imbalance. Counteract this with things like broth, multi-vitamins, multi-minerals, and foods rich in electrolytes like sodium, magnesium and potassium.

Thirdly, eat more fat. We've already discussed the need to get at least 70– 75 percent of your calories from fat, but this is especially important as you initially start the diet. At this early stage, people are often still prone to resisting fatty foods, which only serves to slow down the transition. So help speed up your transition by putting butter and bacon on everything, plopping some heavy cream into your tea or coffee, and eating fatty meals.

Fourthly, make sure that you don't eat too much protein. As discussed earlier, excess protein is converted into glucose which will only serve to slow down your transition. Don't fall for the stereotypical notion that a diet means nibbling on tuna rolls and chicken breast.

All in all, don't give up if you experience symptoms of the keto flu. Push through it. Also, to help alleviate symptoms, make sure that you drink heaps of water, keep your electrolyte levels up, and eat less protein and more fat.

Eventually, you'll experience feelings of euphoria, a burst in energy, and fat loss. You will also notice that your urine develops a strong smell and your mouth develops a bit of a metallic taste. From this, you'll know that it's working!

# Mistake #10: Confused Carb Counting

A problem that many on the ketogenic diet encounter is this: Total carbs or net carbs? What really counts?

While total carbs count everything, net carbs don't count fibre. The reasoning behind so many people counting only net carbs — also known as available carbohydrates — is that there is a belief that dietary fibre has no effect on blood sugar and that our body is unable to derive any calories from it.

So is this true?

Well, not completely. Fibre can be broken down into two main components: Insoluble fibre and soluble fibre. And as the name "*soluble* fibre" indicates, fibre does actually count — at least some of it. So while, yes, insoluble fibre can't be absorbed and doesn't impact blood sugar or ketosis, this is not the case for soluble fibre.

The FDA (Food and Drug Administration) found that our bodies can indeed derive calories from soluble fibre. Studies have also found that soluble fibre can potentially increase blood sugar and thus hinder or prevent ketosis. For this reason, some experts recommend counting total carbs instead of net carbs.

That being said, even some of the experts disagree on whether or not to include fibre when counting carbohydrate intake. Dr. Volek and Dr. Phinney count total carbs and suggest that 50 grams of total carbs will induce ketosis. Depending on fibre content, 50 grams of total carbs should be roughly 20–35 grams of net carbs. It is worth noting that for most people on the ketogenic diet, this approach works.

Dr. Westman also counts total carbs, however he suggests that you should be aiming for 20 grams of total carbs per day.

Overall, it seems that the world's leading low-carb experts count total fibre, not net fibre. A mistake that some people make when embarking on the ketogenic diet is to count net carbs and, as a result, unknowingly affect their blood sugar and hinder or prevent ketosis.

# Mistake #11: Quick to Quit

Among the most common mistakes that those new to the ketogenic diet make is to quit too quickly. This is often the result of unrealistic expectations and people looking for a quick fix. While the ketogenic diet is certainly one of, if not the most, effective of diets, you won't be dropping a pound every half an hour. It doesn't eliminate obesity overnight.

Rather than thinking of the ketogenic diet as a quick-fix diet, think of it as a lifestyle change. You won't reap any long-term benefits if you just "go keto" to drop a few pounds before going straight back to what you were eating.

Although the "keto flu" only lasts several days, it generally takes several weeks for your body to fully adapt to burning fat instead of carbohydrate-derived glucose. For this reason, it is important to be patient when starting out. It is equally important to make sure that you are strict when it comes to sticking to the diet.

So don't fall for the trap of having unrealistic expectations of overnight transformation and then promptly quitting when they don't materialize. Rather, a safe amount for someone who has a lot of weight to lose would be around 1.5–2.5 pounds per week. Someone with less weight to lose, say, 10–20 pounds, should aim for 0.5–1 pound per week.

Just remember that weight loss takes time. Though cliche, it's a marathon and not a sprint. Also, it's important to keep in mind that some people are able to lose weight faster than others. So — as much as I hate to say it — have realistic expectations. For example, 1–2 pounds a week is a realistic goal, while hoping to lose 10 pounds within the fortnight is unrealistic.

When it comes to weight loss, it is easy to get discouraged and quit when expectations that are borderline physically impossible don't materialize. Diligently stay with it for the long haul and you will achieve your goals and reap all the rewards.

# Mistake #12: Exercising Correctly

If you're striving for weight loss on the ketogenic diet, it is important to make sure that you are exercising correctly. Doing too much exercise or not doing any exercise are both counterproductive for weight loss.

One of the most common false beliefs about exercise that hold people back from achieving long-term weight loss is not utilizing exercise effectively. They view exercise as a method of burning calories. This is like selling a rental property to make money. Yes, you will make some money from the initial sale, that's it. Similarly, when people get off the treadmill, that's it. They stop burning calories as soon as they stop.

There is a better way to get the most out of your exercise and achieve long-term weight loss. You will keep burning calories indefinitely, even after you've stopped working out. Just like a rental property keeps bringing in rent indefinitely.

How?

While light cardio exercise (such as running) has great benefits for the heart and brain, weight training is often better for long-term weight loss. This is because weight training grows muscle, and muscles burn fat — even when you're not at the gym. A person with more muscle burns more fat than someone who doesn't have as much muscle. Just as a Ferrari burns more fuel than a little Toyota — even when driving at the same speed.

Studies have also found excessive exercise to lead to increased appetites and thus overeating. Likewise, doing little to no exercise will yield no results either. Furthermore, you're much more likely to continue exercising after the initial boost of enthusiasm is gone if your daily workout isn't three hours long.

Keep in mind that in the beginning of your diet, your physical performance might suffer. Just go easy and allow your body time to adapt and adjust — once you begin running on fat rather than carbs, your performance will recover. That being said, it is important that you don't neglect to exercise. The body's natural response to weight loss is to conserve energy (and thus hinder your weight loss efforts). Exercise counteracts this.

All in all, exercise, just don't overdo it. Also make sure that you include weight training in your exercise routine to ensure long-term weight loss.

# Mistake #13: Fantastic Fibre

An easy mistake to make when starting out on the ketogenic diet is to not get enough fibre.

Meat doesn't have fibre. Dairy doesn't have fibre. It's easy to see how one can end up not getting enough fibre. The problem with this is that if you don't get enough fibre, you can end up with constipation and even hemorrhoids.

Compared to carbohydrates, fat and protein are not as easy to digest and pass through your system. So it is super important to make sure that you get enough fibre.

The best sources of natural fibre include vegetables, berries, and nuts. That being said, these foods also contain a small amount of carbs, meaning that these foods are often avoided. In this case, the best solution is to take a fibre supplement.

Another problem those on the ketogenic diet encounter is poor gut health. This is the result of a high intake of animal protein (e.g. fatty foods) and low intake of indigestible fibre (e.g. fruits and vegetables high in fibre). This can result in having inflammatory gut bacteria that release chemicals which elevate inflammation and increase the buildup of plaque.

In addition to increasing fibre intake, such as through a supplement, you eliminate the risk of inflammatory gut bacteria by eating probiotic foods such as kefir, kimchi, yogurt, and sauerkraut.

Finally, aside from vegetables, fruit and supplements, chia seeds are a great source of fibre. And not only are they a great source of fibre, but they're also high in fat!

Moreover, 75 percent of the fibre in chia seeds is insoluble. This means that unless you completely overdose on them, you shouldn't need to worry too much about their carbs. That being said, it is nonetheless always a good idea keep track of your dietary intake to make sure that you stay on track and reap the full rewards of ketosis.

# Mistake #14: Beer Belly

A mistake made by some is to regularly drink alcohol. There are several reasons why regularly drinking alcohol can prevent you from achieving or maintaining ketosis and turning your body into a fat burning machine.

Firstly, alcoholic drinks contain carbohydrates. Some people don't seem to get the fact that alcohol is a big contributor to weight gain. The term "beer belly" doesn't exist for no reason.

Secondly, alcohol becomes the body's choice of fuel when ingested. Your body won't even sugar as energy if there's alcohol. What this means is that your body will stop burning fat. It won't even burn carbohydrates (i.e. sugar). So by drinking alcohol, you are literally preventing yourself from burning fat and losing weight.

Thirdly, alcohol messes with the body's hormonal balance, making weight loss more difficult.

So while you might be tempted to reassure yourself that a few beers here and there or a glass of wine every other day can't do any harm, the reality is that this could be what is causing your weight loss plateau.

The best solution is to try to cut it out completely.

# Mistake #15: Endless Eating

Just because ketosis means that your body starts burning fat for energy, that does not mean that you should eat as much as you possibly can. People make the mistake of thinking that they can eat a ton of food and that as long as they don't eat carbs, it'll be okay.

Put simply, that is just not true. By eating too much and/or too often, you hinder weight loss.

The simple solution is this: If you are no longer hungry, stop eating. This is not only true for standard diets, but is of even more importance when it comes to low-carb, high-fat diets. This is because food that are high in fat are also much higher in calories. Overeating high-fat foods gives you far more calories than overeating on a normal, low-fat diet.

Luckily, once you achieve ketosis you will find yourself far less hungry. In fact, you will probably find yourself forgetting to eat for hours and hours on end. This is because it takes longer for the body to break down fat and use it for energy. So you can have a high-fat breakfast and then find that you go through the rest of the day without feeling at all hungry. In fact, it's not uncommon for those on the ketogenic diet to admit that they actually do regularly intermittent fasting — without even realizing!

Another reason that the ketogenic diet leaves you forgetting to eat is that your body is full of fat. Pinch some skin on your belly or thigh and you'll realize that your next meal is pre-installed! When your body is used to burning carbohydrates (i.e. sugar) for energy, you typically find yourself wanting breakfast, morning tea, lunch, afternoon tea, dinner, and supper. Not only is this because it takes less time for the body turn carbohydrates into energy, but also because — unlike fat — your body isn't filled with them.

Imagine we have two garbage trucks. One of the trucks burns diesel for fuel. The other garbage truck burns garbage for fuel. Obviously the diesel-powered truck represents a high-carb eater that burns carbs for energy, while the garbage-powered truck represents a ketogenic dieter who burns fat for energy.

Which truck is going to finish the day with the least garbage? The answer is pretty clear, is it not? Obviously the garbage truck that's been burning garbage all day long is going to finish with the least garbage!

Now let's switch things up a little. Imagine if the diesel-powered garbage truck went and emptied rubbish bins in ordinary suburban streets. That's about one rubbish bin every 60 feet. The garbage-powered truck, however, goes into the city and empties the bins of high-rise apartment buildings. Rather than one rubbish bin every 60 feet, it's probably closer to a hundred bins every 60 feet!

In this new example, obviously the diesel-powered truck will end the day with less rubbish. Even though the garbage-powered truck has literally been burning rubbish all day long, it has consumed so much rubbish that it could not burn it all fast enough.

The same thing happens if you overeat. So, yes, you burn fat for energy in ketosis. However, if you overeat, your body is going to be too busy burning the fat that you've eaten to ever even need to worry about burning your body fat. As a result, you will struggle to lose weight.

A big mistake that many people make when starting out on the ketogenic diet is to continue eating as they have in the past on their high-carb diet. When the clock strikes 1 o'clock, they go out and eat. When the clock strikes 8 o'clock, they go have dinner.

It can be hard to break habits, but when you're on the ketogenic diet, ask yourself — are you *really* actually hungry, or are you just eating because the clock tells you it's time for lunch?

One of the reasons your weight loss on the ketogenic diet might be plateauing is that you are eating more than you need. When your body is keto-adapted, you'll find that your hunger is completely zapped. You'll find yourself forgetting to eat and you'll be alert and energized all day long, even while going many hours between meals. Rather than begging you to feed it, your body will be eating away at the pre-installed meals under your skin — stored body fat.

As such, the benefit is twofold. Your body is burning fat *and* your calorie consumption decreases.

So, stop feeling like you need to eat a certain amount of food. Far too many people make the mistake of unknowingly continuing the habit of eating three full meals and two snacks each day. Eat only when you're hungry, not just because the clock tells you to. If you overeat, the body won't get a chance to burn all that fat you want to lose.

# Mistake #16: Neglecting MCTs

Another common mistake that people make when starting out on the ketogenic diet is to neglect MCTs. MCT stands for medium-chain triglycerides. Triglyceride is pretty much just a fancy word for fat.

MCTs are are a special type of fat that are extremely easy to digest. Most fats — LCTs, long-chain triglycerides — take longer to digest because, as the name suggests, they are longer. Medium-chain fats are easier and quicker to break down than long-chain fats.

The fact that almost all fats are of the long-chain variety (i.e. LCTs), it's not uncommon for people starting out on the ketogenic diet — a diet that is almost all fat —

to feel cravings for carbohydrates and the quick energy they provide.

So what's the solution?

MCTs! As these fats are very, very quickly broken down, they can provide you with a quick energy boost.

The only downside, however, is that MCTs are extremely rare in most foods. In fact, they are pretty much only found in coconuts. As such, the best way to take advantage of MCTs is to get a bunch of coconut oil to use when needed. You can chuck some in your tea or coffee of a morning or before exercising.

If you find yourself being overcome with fatigue or brain fog for the first few weeks as your body fully adapts to your new diet, make sure that you're not neglecting MCTs.

Furthermore, another great benefit of MCTs are that they have been shown to actually help you to burn more fat!

Sound too good to be true?

As opposed to other common dietary components, MCTs are sent straight to the liver. While most dietary fats (i.e. LCTs) have to go through your lymph system before reaching the liver and becoming ketones, this is not true for MCTs.

MCTs enter the liver directly. Straight away. No detours.

What this means for you is that your body is able to quickly produce ketone bodies and boost your energy levels.

There are also countless — well, around 26 or more, to be exact — studies that reveal that MCTs show potential in not only maintaining a healthy weight but in actually decreasing fat storage.

And as if MCTs don't already have enough benefits, they also leave you feeling full — even more so than ordinary fats (i.e. LCTs). This obviously means that you are less likely to overeat, and so you'll also be getting the benefits of eating less!

If you are looking to make the most of MCTs, a great source is *Bulletproof Brain Octane Oil* — a condensed form of coconut oil. It's so rich in MCTs that you would literally need 18 tablespoons of ordinary coconut oil to match that found in a single tablespoon of Brain Octane.

Furthermore, MCTs help fuel brain function. Not only do MCTs quickly produce ketones in the body, providing the brain with energy, but — even better — MCTs can instantly be used by the brain for energy. Instantly!

How?

They can pass straight through the brain-blood barrier. This gives you that much needed quick boost of mental clarity, allowing you to perform at your best. MCTs also enhance and boost ketone production as well as stabilize blood sugar.

A problem that many people starting out on the ketogenic diet struggle with is an initial lack of energy. While your body will adapt from deriving most of its energy from glucose to deriving most of its energy from ketones within a week or so (after the keto flu), it can take up to a full month for your body to fully adapt.

During these several weeks, MCTs can be of great help. Moreover, even once your body fully adapts to burning fat, you might still find yourself occasionally craving the quick boost of energy that carbs provide. Rather than messing up ketosis by eating too many carbs, go for the quick energy boost provided by MCTs.

You can incorporate MCTs into your diet by chucking some coconut oil or Brain Octane into your salad dressing, coffee, sports drink, or smoothie. Heck, you can even make some mayonnaise with it — an egg, ¾ cup of olive oil, ¼ cup of Brain Octane, 3 teaspoons of lemon or lime juice, and a pinch of salt.

All in all, make sure to you're not neglecting MCTs. MCTs can also provide a quick boost in energy without kicking you out of ketosis or sending your blood sugar levels sky-high.

# Conclusion

When starting out on the ketogenic diet, many people make mistakes. Almost all of these mistakes can easily be avoided when you are able to identify them and correct them. Hopefully this book has provided you with that knowledge — whether you're just starting out, struggling to achieve ketosis, struggling to maintain ketosis, or are plateauing and looking to maximise the benefits of ketosis.

As you will likely want to be able to quickly refer back to the solutions to these common mistakes in the future, I have created a "cheat sheet" for you at the end that summarises the key points and information discussed in the book.

To conclude, I earnestly hope that you have found benefit in the information provided. That you have a deeper and more thorough understanding of the ketogenic diet, how it works, and how to maximise results. That you are now better equipped to reap the rewards of ketosis, turn yourself into a fat-burning machine, and achieve and *exceed* your weight loss goals.

Best wishes and good luck!

# Cheat Sheet

Here is a quick cheat sheet for you in case you ever need to refer back to any mistakes you might be making if you're struggling to achieve ketosis or are seeing your weight loss results plateau.

## Mistake #1: Scale Surveillance

Don't obsess over the number on the scale. It is a very poor indicator of your overall progress. Furthermore, you can be losing fat but you wouldn't even know — at least by looking at your scale — because you might also be gaining muscle. If you want to keep track of your progress, use other methods. Your general feelings of wellbeing, how your clothes fit, your waistline, your body fat percentage, and so on.

## Mistake #2: Protein Problems

Far too many on the ketogenic diet eat too much protein. Aim for only around 20–25 percent of your calories to come from protein. Excess protein is converted into glucose which can end up hindering or preventing ketosis. Instead, eat more fat. Aim for approximately 75 percent fat, 20 percent protein, and 5 percent carbohydrates.

### Mistake #3: Crazy for Carbs

Carbohydrates can hide in unexpected places. Low fat milk? Bananas? Nuts? They all have carbohydrates. Furthermore, many pre-packaged products labeled "low-carb" are often higher in carbohydrates than they would have you believe. They're also full of additives, sweeteners, and preservatives that mess up your hormones and can hinder your fat loss aspirations.

### Mistake #4: Electrolyte Errors

Make sure you get enough sodium (i.e. salt). When you abandon carbohydrates, your kidneys start dumping lots of sodium which will leave you with headaches, cramps, feelings of fatigue and general unwellness if not counteracted. So put salt on your food, drink broth, and makes sure that you get at least 3 grams of sodium each day.

<u>Mistake #5: Fat Fears</u>

Abandon your deeply held fear of fat. I know you've been told ever since you were a child that fat is bad, however this is only the case if your eat lots of carbohydrates. When you abandon carbohydrates, your body needs a different source of energy — fat. If you don't eat enough fat when on a low-carb diet, you are basically starving yourself. So eat up!

If you're still concerned about fat, there are countless studies that show not only that the ketogenic diet is safe in the long-term, but also that heart disease, bad cholesterol and the like are caused not by fat, but by other factors such as inactivity and — especially — high carbohydrate intake. That being said, if you continue eating high-carb *and* high-fat, then you are putting yourself in a dangerous situation. Eat no more than 50 grams of carbohydrates a day and you've no scientific reasons to fear fat.

## Mistake #6: The Negotiator

If you are not all in on the ketogenic diet, then do not do it. Remaining somewhere between high-carb and high-fat will damage your health and only serve to increase your weight. The ketogenic diet is not for the half-hearted or the uncommitted. Either go all in or don't do it at all. You will not reap the health and fat-burning rewards of ketosis if you half-ass it. You must be 100 percent committed.

## Mistake #7: Fake Food

Eat real food. Avoid pre-packaged meals and processed foods, including health bars. Take the mindset of eating not "food," but "ingredients." Things such as meat and veggies. Often pre-packaged foods get by with deceptive labeling which only counts certain types of sugars and carbohydrates, leading to you actually ending up with more than you realize. Furthermore, they are also full of preservatives, additives, sweeteners, and chemicals that can mess up your hormones and hinder (or even prevent!) your efforts to achieve and/or maintain ketosis.

Eat real food.

## Mistake #8: Friendly Fats and Unfriendly Fats

There are good fats and bad fats. Don't make the mistake of consuming the bad fats.

Good fats include saturated fats and polyunsaturated fats. This encompasses things from Greek yogurt to olive oil and avocados. Refer to inside the book for a more extensive list.

Bad fats are mostly trans fats. The most common source of trans fats are vegetable oils. Avoid any products with trans fats, such as margarine. Instead of margarine, for example, go for the good fats such as that of grass-fed butter.

## Mistake #9: Flu Fighters

When starting out on the ketogenic diet, most people get what has become known as the "keto flu." Symptoms include headaches, fatigue, nausea, and so on. Push through it. It generally only lasts a few days. This just goes to show that the diet is working! Your body is in the process of transforming into a fat-burning machine.

That being said, you can help alleviate the symptoms by eating more fat and less carbs and protein. Also, make sure that you drink lots and lots of water. It is also super important to make sure that you get enough electrolytes — sodium and potassium. You can take care of this by adding salt to your food or drinking broth for salt, and taking some supplements or multivitamins for the potassium.

While all this will help to alleviate the symptoms, it will not completely cure you. For this reason, it is best to start the diet on a weekend so that you are able to rest.

Once you get through it a few days later, you'll be feeling more refreshed than you've felt in years and have an abundance of energy. So push through it! Don't quit!

Mistake #10: Confused Carb Counting

Don't make the mistake of thinking that fibre does not count as a carbohydrate. The reality is that there are two components to fibre: Insoluble fibre and soluble fibre. In other words, fibre can still be absorbed and can push you over the carbohydrate threshold and prevent you from reaching ketosis.

Make sure you do not exceed 50 grams of *total* carbs each day. If that doesn't get you into full-blown ketosis (which it should), you might want to follow the advice of some other leading low-carb medical experts who suggest that you should aim for 20 grams of *total* carbs.

Mistake #11: Quick to Quit

Don't be quick to quit. The ketogenic diet is not a "quick fix" nor will it lead to an overnight transformation. Rather, the ketogenic diet is a *lifestyle*.

Moreover, it can take your body up to a full month for it to fully adapt to burning fat rather than glucose (i.e. carbs). Persist and don't give up too early. Quitters never win and winners never quit!

Mistake #12: Exercising Correctly

Exercising is an important part of weight loss. That being said, over exerting yourself can also have negative effects. Find a sustainable exercise routine. Find balance and stick to it consistently.

Also, it is important to incorporate weight training into your exercise routine if you want to achieve long-term weight loss. Weight training helps to build muscle, and muscle burns fat. The more muscle, the more fat you burn. Conversely, cardio exercise — such as going for a run or bike ride — only burns calories during the actual exercise. Growing muscle will continue to burn calories and fat indefinitely, even when you're not exercising.

## Mistake #13: Fantastic Fibre

A lack of dietary fibre can lead to constipation, hemorrhoids, poor gut health, and internal inflammation. While you may not be able to get natural fibre from fruits due to the carbohydrate content in most fruits, do not neglect dietary fibre. You can try foods that are high in fibre like chia seeds, or, even better, you can take fibre supplements. Make sure to keep that fibre intake up!

## Mistake #14: Beer Belly

Regular alcohol intake can prevent you from reaping the rewards of full-blown ketosis. Seriously. Not only is alcohol high in carbohydrates (the term "beer belly" exists for a reason!), but when alcohol is ingested, it becomes the body's energy source. In other words, your body will stop burning glucose, it will stop burning fat, and will instead be burning alcohol for energy. As such, by drinking alcohol, you are literally stopping your body from burning fat. So cut out the alcohol, or at the very least, don't drink it regularly.

## Mistake #15: Endless Eating

Just because you are on a low-carb diet, that doesn't mean you can eat as much food as you want. The whole point of the ketogenic diet is to get your body burning body fat. However, if you eat heaps of food, then your body has no reason to burn body fat! Overeating will prevent you from burning body fat and losing weight.

## Mistake #16: Neglecting MCTs

As fat takes a long time to burn and be converted into energy, you might find yourself craving the quick energy boost that carbs give you. Don't succumb to this desire and end up sabotaging ketosis. Instead, make the most of MCTs!

MCTs are a form of fat that is very quickly broken down and turned into energy. They are found in coconut oil and products derived from coconut oil such as Brain Octane. If you're looking for a quick energy boost, MCTs are the way to go.

Made in the USA
San Bernardino, CA
04 June 2018